JUICING RECIPES
for Newbies

Ana Ortega

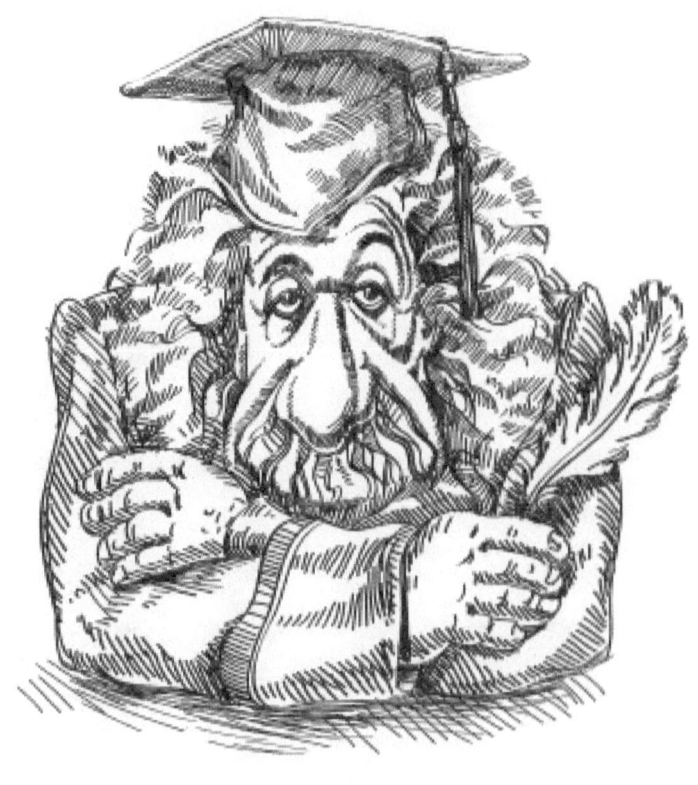

*Nothing will benefit human health and
increase chances for survival of Life on Earth
as much as the evolution to a vegetarian diet –*

Albert Einstein

CONTENTS

Preface
Why Juicing
Warnings
Tool Time
The Newbie Healing shopping list

Juices!

PREFACE

I am passionate about health and finding healthy ways of nurturing my body optimize its performance and assist the cell renewal. Moreover, I am fully dedicated to help improve the health and habits of anyone and everyone looking for change. And what is most important, Sometime ago I discovered that my life purpose is to inspire individuals like you, help you dream and believe that those dreams can be accomplished with a bit of determination, a great dose of dedication and directed actions.

Intention is everything in life. And after the overwhelming success of Vegan Recipes for Newbie's, witnessing how I have changed the lives and bodies of thousands for the better and continue inspiring many others with my Life Coaching services, I am committed to help you in your quest to IMPROVE YOURSELF and make you materialize your dreams. And for an unknown reason, I SIMPLY KNOW that together, you and I, we can make this journey a fun and successful one. So, let me help you and help yourself transform your body as you progress in YOUR journey of Self-discovery and embrace new level of UNDERSTANDING.

Start your day every morning looking at yourself in the mirror and seeing yourself as a creative individual with CREATIVE POWERS. You are more than a body; you are more than your name and your education. You are much more than your income, that the city you leave in. You are a magnificent creation whose purpose is to find real fulfillment.

Life is SIMPLE. We complicate our worlds by the inability of making our own decisions and allowing others to live and control our lives for ourselves. I am determined to show you how you can achieve your optimal health state in a very simple way. GOING BACK TO BASICS- eating the products Mother Nature kindly and gratefully gave us and making great use of the technology we, the human mind has created- Yes, we have created technology nowadays using that creative power I am talking about here! And,Yes! I am referring to the fantastic JUICE MAKER!

We are not beings living a spiritual experience; we are spirit having a human experience. Our body is an instrument for the spirit to act and express itself towards the accomplishment of ideas that were at first generated from formless thought substance. Our body and mind create the world we live in. A strong mind requires of a strong and healthy body. Get it? No? Then I suggest that you go back to the start, re- read these concepts until you do because then and only then you will have a clear picture about how this book can help you achieve the goal you have established for yourself at a physical and mental level- whether if it is to lose that extra weight, or feel more energetic and dynamic. Whatever the goal is, you have decided to get on hold of this book, and that is a great start! So, Congratulations! And let's continue the great work!

Realize that when you facing unwanted situations in your life, may they be sickness, may it be lack of confidence and poor self image or may it be something else completely different, you do get to choose how you react to these unwanted circumstances and by doing so, you will then control the extent of how much you will hurt at a mental and physical level. If you choose to respond irrationally or by being over sensitive and taking things too personally, I can guarantee that you will suffer.

However, only with controlled ACTIONS, PERSISTENCE and JOY you can turn your present circumstances around and ACCOMPLISH anything you desire.

ANYTHING! So that one day, those old days would be a distant memory, the dark side of the bright life you now live, as the night is to the day, as the black is to white. Take control of your life, and take it now. I am here to help you all the way through.

So... THE BIG WHY...Why Juicing?

I was introduced to juicing when I was twelve years old. I will always remember the day my dad brought home the first juicer and started blending everything green he could get his hands on. At first, I found juicing too extravagant and complicated for my taste. But dad would never give up (now you know where my stubbornness comes from!) And he would continue blending and mixing veggies and fruits in search for the perfect juice. So now, after over twenty years drinking vegetable juices on a regular basis, I am not only hocked but also completely convinced freshly made vegetable juices play an important role in having a radiant body and mind and energetic life, as well as a truly optimal health.

This time I decided to share my experience with you and create a very simple recipe book and not a textbook. Again, I am keeping things simple and straightforward for you so that you can start benefiting from making fresh vegetable juices from day one.

 If you need details on scientific research studies, then I suggest you give away this book because it is not for you.

There is however something I can tell you. I wrote this

recipe book to share with you my favorite vegetable juices- the ones and only those one that I know that really work for the busy modern person on the go who is looking to embrace a healthy lifestyle, without compromising in taste nor breaking the bank account.

As I busy entrepreneur, self confessed food addict and Life coach I am, I wrote this simple juicing book taking into account the three most important things in my life: HEALTH, FOOD, SELF-APRECIATION.

Media and health experts bombard us recommending eating our 6-8 daily servings of vegetables and fruits, which, honestly, it can be really a challenge to do if you have a busy lifestyle and you are "on the go". It is here where juicing becomes a friendly helper in achieving this recommended goal.

The beauty about juicing lies also that you can start with right away and get results in no time. Your body will benefit from it from the moment you get started.

Be wary, I am not saying that you need to go on a fast one week juicing diet where all you do is juicing. I am simply asking you to start integrating freshly made vegetable and fruit juices into your diet until it becomes your habit! If you are thinking of going on a fasting diet, then please please please pretty please with sugar on top, consult with your doctor. Your health is your biggest wealth; promise me right here right now to take care of yourself!

I suggest making green juices first thing in the morning and drinking them in an empty stomach, so that the goodness of the vitamins and minerals of those veggies penetrates your blood stream reaching and nurturing your cells.

Green juices are the breakfast of the champions! They are delicious, fully customizable as you can use seasonal vegetables and fruits and anything green at hand. You can drink it at home or when in rush make it "to go", it requires no cooking whatsoever and yet provides you with plenty of nutrients to start your day off on the right foot. I could list hundreds reasons why you should juice your greens. But I will leave it opt to you to try and experience every and all of them and increase the list of benefits.

Don't let their sometimes-funny rainbow of colors deceive you. STAY FOCUS, you CAN do IT. Stay away from all sort of negativity and those who will find an excuse not to get you in the right track. Yes, I am talking about those friends and family members, unwilling to try new things themselves and afraid of being forced change simply because you have decided you are improving yourself. They will pour on you their fears and will try to prevent you from trying. They are likely to come up with excuses and old myths such as: *"Cleaning the juicer is a job on its own! "*, *"But What about the fiber?"*, *"Your stomach is going to be messed up drinking all those greens"*.

The important thing for you to know is that first, you ARE NOT on a fasting diet, you are still having and enjoying your nice lunch and dinners and likely to be WITH THEM– do check out *Vegan Recipes for Newbies* for some inspiration – and secondly when you juice, yes it is true that you don't get the fiber that's in whole fruits and vegetables. BUT Juicing machines do extract the juice and leave behind the pulp, which has all the fiber. If you really do wish to add extra fiber into your diet, you can always add some of the pulp back into the juice or us it in your cooking to fortify your meals or to bake wonderful cakes!

And let me highlight for you some other reasons that you can give them:

- You will gain vitality and stamina

- Increased mental clarity

- Better sleep

- Improve self image

- Reduce cell inflammation – those morning puffy eyes will be long forgotten the moment you start juicing!

- Anti-aging properties

- Oxygenate your body thanks to the chlorophyll in the green vegetables

- Efficient abortion of minerals such as potassium and Vitamins such as Vitamin C and Bs.

- Vitamin C rich fruits and vegetables will help replenish your skin's vitamin C stores and enhance its natural beauty.

- Aids in maintenance of healthy and lustrorous hair.

- May help in joint flexibility; prevent cataracts, and macular degeneration.

- Body fat reduction

- Improve your metabolism

- Will increase the number of blood cells (combat anemia)

- Hydrate your body easily, quickly and stay better nourished

- Removes toxins from the body

- Purifies the liver

- The increased Irons supply will benefit your heart tissue

- Counter disorders in blood sugar, which calms cravings, and food related addictive patterns.

- Eliminates body odor

- Improves nasal drainage

- Increases milk production

- It relieves inflammation (throat, etc..)

- Relieves ulcers

- Eliminates cold or mucus

- Destroy bacteria from wounds

- Mitigates the pain of hemorrhoids

- Revitalizes vascular system in the legs

- Reduces pain from inflammation

- Improves varicose veins

- It purifies the intestines and colon

- Helps fight hepatitis

- Help hemophilia

- Help us improve asthma disorders

- The sores heal faster

What more reasons?

Did you know that 95% of the vitamins and enzymes our bodies need are found in the juice of raw fruits and vegetables? Did you know that drinking daily green juices raises nutrient rich liquid sun goodness straight into your blood? And did you know that every one of us completely regenerate our own skin every 7 days? Would it be amazing if we could find a way to lie down a great foundation for these new baby cells to develop?

WARNING

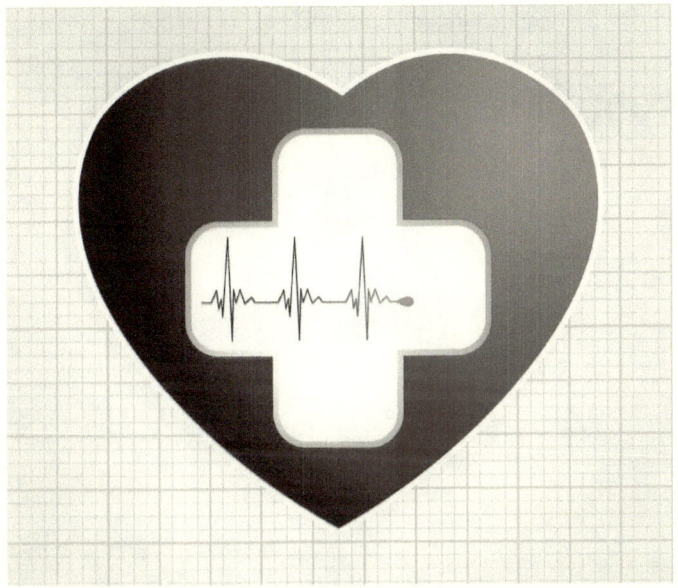

While certainly you can make fruit juices, if you are overweight, have currently any health problems such as high blood pressure or cholesterol or diabetes; please do consult with your doctor before embracing juicing. It is likely that you will be asked to limit your fruit intake to have these problems under control.

An alternative you can ask your doctor is about citric such as lemons, kiwis and limes due to the low fructose content. Not to mention, they are also great as a way to balance the bitter taste of some dark green leafed vegetables.

Also, It is important to note that vegetable juices have very little protein and almost no fat, and alone should not be considered as a complete food. So the juicing I am proposing here in this simple guide should be used as food supplement and not as their only food!

TOOL TIME!

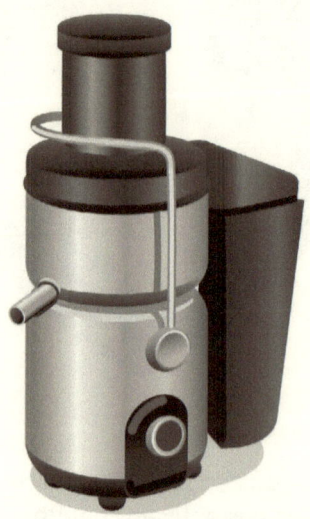

That is right! Call it Juice Maker, Juice Extractor, Juicer... You can call it a hundreds different ways and it is all you need to get started. Your very own toy!

And I suggest that you invest in a nice one as you are going to use it a lot. Think about it as a pal in your quest to a better version of you.

You can get a decent juicer from prices starting at 200 dollars. PREPARATION is key in anything you do. So do your research and buy the one that you really like as your ROI (Return on Investment) is going to blow your mind away in no time!

And whatever your schedule is please remember to clean your juicer after using it to avoid giving birth to new forms of life. Yes, I am talking about contaminating the extractor leftovers with mold.

BUT

DO NOT let this minor task put you off- And believe me when I tell you that your mind will find excuses just to stop juicing a this point. When it happens just think or say out loud: STOP THAT, or NEXT and STAY FOCUS. Think of the reason you got started in the first place. YOU CAN DO IT.

Dot not quit! You have the willpower within your self to rise above your circumstances

THE NEWBIE HEALING SHOPPING LIST

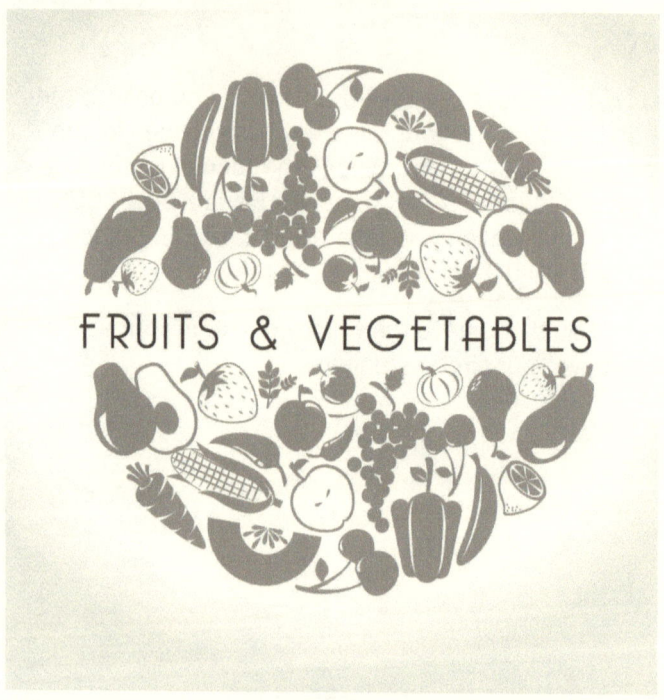

Here are my top vegetable picks

Celery
Spinach
Kale
Chard
Lettuce
Carrots
Cucumber
Parsley

Fennel
Radish
Turnip
Sweet potato (skin on)
Broccoli
Cabbage
Tomatoes
Eggplant
Peppers – I absolutely adore the taste of red peppers
Beet
Mint/ Ginger to spice things up a little more

And...

Here are my top Fruit choice

Pears
Apples
Watermelon (rind removed)
Melon
Orange (peeled)
Pineapple (peeled)
Apricots and Peach (pitted)
Cranberries
Dragon fruit
Kiwi
Berries

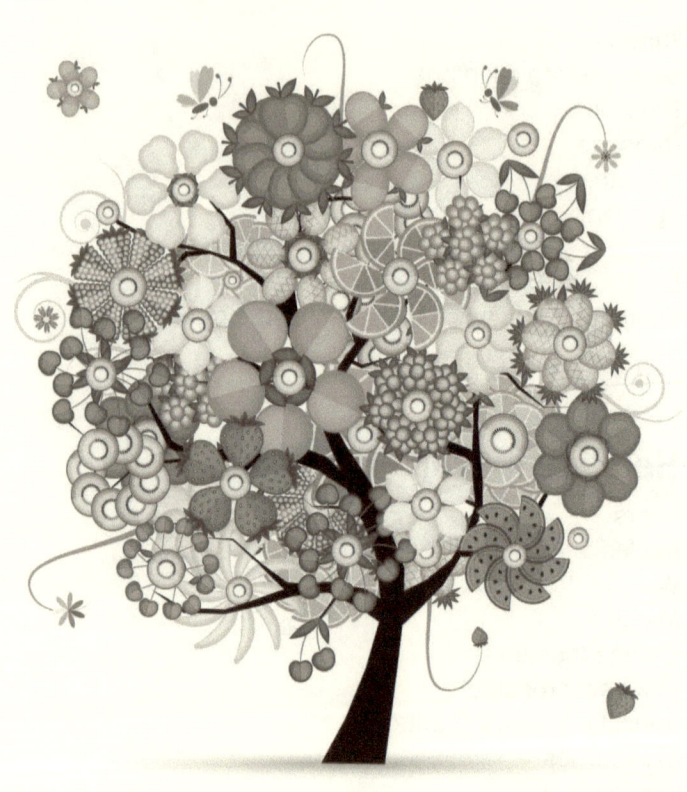

JUICES

This is where the fun part starts! I have included in this simple guide a 100 of my favorite recipes. Each one of them comes with a daily message aimed at reaching at your subconscious directly- whether you understand the message or not, it is unimportant. What it matters is that the system is infallible. It works!

These are 100 juicing recipes will help you achieve success in all areas of your life because you are working on yourself from within. So be prepared to be amazed, be ready to receive gracefully your new health, and feel better at a personal level.

An improved version of yourself will expand further than you ever imagined you could have reached in this lifetime. But most importantly, feel free to express yourself. BE courageous, BE fearless, BE yourself. BE creative. You really cannot go wrong here. It is all about experimenting, creating and have fun all the way through. BE Joy!

BE something TODAY, right HERE, right NOW!

DIRECTIONS

Couldn't get any easier...

STEP 1 Wash and prepare your ingredients. Turn on your juicer to the slowest setting and juice and serve immediately.

STEP 2 Give the juice a good stir

Please note: You can store juice for up to 24 hours. Pour it into an airtight container, leaving as little airspace as possible to reduce oxidation, and store it in the refrigerator.

Next challenge please!!! ....

**Enjoy the day ahead.
Do what you love,
and Love what you do!**

**Smile, Dance, Love, laugh and LIVE.
Be grateful. Be YOU**

JUICES

Detox bliss I

Ingredients:

2 small heads of bok choy
1 lemon (peeled)
1 cucumber (unpeeled)
A little piece of fresh ginger (peeled)
1/2 pineapple (peeled)

Detox bliss II

Ingredients:

1 cucumber (unpeeled)
A handful of spinaches
1 pear

Youth fountain

Ingredients:

4 kale leaves
1 lemon (peeled)
1 cucumber (unpeeled)
a little piece of fresh ginger (peeled)
1 green apple (unpeeled)

Glow, Baby Glow

Ingredients:

½ mango (peeled)
1/2 lemon (peeled)
1 cucumber (unpeeled)
Handful parsley

Morning wake up I

Ingredients:

1 green apple (unpeeled)
1 cucumber (unpeeled)
1 celery stick
½ lemon (peeled)

Morning wake up II

Ingredients:

1 green apple (unpeeled)
1 cucumber (unpeeled)
1 celery stick
½ lemon (peeled)
1 Yellow pepper

Love handles? No thank you very much!

Ingredients:

2 medium carrots (unpeeled)
1 cucumber (unpeeled)
1 red pepper
1 lemon (peeled)

Look at me NOW I

Ingredients:

1 green apple (unpeeled)
1 cucumber (unpeeled)
1 celery stick
½ lemon (peeled)
a handful of spring greens

Pure consciousness!

Ingredients:

1 green apple (unpeeled)
1 cucumber (unpeeled)
2 large carrots
½ lemon (peeled)
1 large red pepper

Look at me NOW II

Ingredients:

1 green pear (unpeeled)
1 cucumber (unpeeled)
2 celery stick
2 kiwis

Summer mood

Ingredients:

1/2 cup (120 ml) cold water
1 orange (peeled)
1 red apple
1 slice of fresh pineapple
1 medium carrot

Citrus Carrot Juice

Ingredients:

1/2 cup (120 ml) cold water
4 medium carrots
1 lemon or piece of fresh ginger (peeled)

Morning Glow

Ingredients:

200g fresh spinach leaves
1 randarin orange
1 large cucumber
Mint leaves

Strong hearts

Ingredients:

1 cup of green grapes
1 large pear
1 cucumber
100 g kale

Love my me

Ingredients:

20 strawberries
3 large carrots
1/2 Lemon
1/2 red pepper

Love my body

Ingredients:

1 slice of fresh pineapple
½ beet Root
3 carrots
1 orange (peeled)
½ red cabbage
1 lemon (peeled)

Happy Buddha

Ingredients:

1 green apple
1 pear
2 carrots
1 celery stick
1 lemon (peeled)
A little piece of turmeric root
A little piece of ginger root

Clear mind

Ingredients:

1 green apple
1 celery stick
a good bunch of baby spinach leaves
1 kale
1 lemon (peeled)
a bunch of fresh parsley

Tropical Madness

Ingredients:

1 mango (peeled and pitted)
1 pineapple (peeled)
1 kale
1 orange (peeled)
A little piece of fresh ginger

Salsa forever

Ingredients:

1 tomato
1 sweet green pepper
1 celery stick
1 red/sweet onion
1 garlic clove
A little tea spoon of cayenne Pepper (spice)

Summer Song

Ingredients:

1 tomato
1 celery stick
1 cucumber
2 carrots
1 sweet green pepper
A bunch of spinach leaves
A bunch of parsley

Exotic punch

Ingredients:

1 pineapple (peeled)
2 kiwis (peeled)
1 pear
1 lime (peeled)
a bunch of mint leaves

Hangover remedy

Ingredients:

1 grapefruit (peeled)
1 small bitter melon (peeled)
1 lemon (peeled)

Wonder Breakfast

Ingredients:

1 green apple
1 cucumber
2 carrots
1 sweet yellow pepper
1 tomato
10 grapes
A bunch of spinaches

Renew me

Ingredients:

1 celery stick
5 green/ white asparagus
A bunch of fresh coriander
½ lemon (peeled)

Goodbye to puffiness

Ingredients:

3 carrots
2 celery sticks
3 large green asparagus

Earthy goodness

Ingredients:

3 large carrots
1 beet root
1 large sweet potato

Tan with kick

Ingredients:

4 carrots
1 green apple
1 lemon (peeled)
a little piece of fresh ginger root

Xray Vision

Ingredients:

4 carrots
½ cabbage
A bunch of parsley
½ lemon (peeled)

Mojo Infusion

Ingredients:

4 carrots
1 green apple
½ lemon (peeled)
2 cloves of garlic (peeled)
a bunch of parsley

Wild and Savage

Ingredients:

20 fresh blackberries
2 pears
1 kiwi (peeled)
A little piece of fresh ginger root
A bunch of peppermint leaves

Touch me

Ingredients:

1 cucumber
1 red apple
1 grapefruit
2 peaches (pitted and with skin)
½ lemon (peeled)

Acne Miracle cure

Ingredients:

1 onion (peeled)
3 carrots
A bunch of parsley
1 lemon (peeled)

Stop & Breath

Ingredients:

200 ml organic coconut water
1 cucumber
1 orange
2 peaches (pitted and with skin)

Fly flu

Ingredients:

3 carrots
6 radishes
1 grapefruit (peeled)
a little piece of fresh ginger

Bang, Bang. Alive!

Ingredients:

1 cucumber
3 celery sticks
1 green apple
a little piece of green ginger
2 limes (peeled)

Midnight green coco

Ingredients:

100 ml organic coconut water
3 celery sticks
A teaspoon of honey

Skinny peach

Ingredients:

1 cucumber
3 peaches (pitted)
3 carrots
1 green apple
½ lemon (peeled)

Full tank please

Ingredients:

1 cucumber
1 yellow pepper
1 pear
20 strawberries
a bunch of fresh peppermint leaves

Forever young

Ingredients:

20-30 black grapes
200 g fresh blackberries
1 kiwi (peeled)
1 lemon (peeled)

Juicy strawberry

Ingredients:

1 cucumber
20 strawberries
1 red pepper
1 grapefruit (peeled)

Wrinkle free potion

Ingredients:

1 medium sugar pumpkin (cut in cubes to fit your juicer)
1 pear
1 orange (peeled)
1 lemon (peeled)
½ teaspoon cinnamon

Boost my mood

Ingredients:

1 celery stick
1 apple
2 carrots
1 Beet root
a bunch of fresh parley

Happiness from Within

Ingredients:

1 carrot
1 cucumber
A bunch of fresh spinach leaves
1 pear
1 lemon (peeled)
a little piece of fresh ginger root

Freedom in a Jar

Ingredients:

1 celery stick
1 cucumber
1 apple
a bunch of fresh spinach leaves
1 lime (peeled)
1 lemon (peeled)
a bunch of fresh parsley

Fitness to go

Ingredients:

1 apple
1 celery stick
1 orange (peeled)
1 lemon (peeled)

Green Tonic

Ingredients:

1 cucumber
1 endive head
1 lettuce
a little piece of fresh ginger root

Bloody Mary

Ingredients:

1 cucumber
1 tomato
1 lemon (peeled)
a bit of salt and pepper to taste
a drop of Tabasco sauce (optional)

Tropical Bomb

Ingredients:

1 cucumber
1 mango (petted)
a bunch of fresh spinach leaves
2 pears
a bunch of fresh mint leaves

Sugar Daddy

Ingredients:

1 cucumber
1 orange (peeled)
4 carrots
1 lemon (peeled)
a bunch of fresh mint leaves

Lime Fizz

Ingredients:

2 pears
2 celery sticks
3 limes (peeled)
a little piece of fresh ginger root

Mediterranean Beauty

Ingredients:

4 carrots
2 oranges (peeled)
5 large strawberries
a bunch of fresh mint leaves

Pink Rum

Ingredients:

1 cucumber
1 red pepper
1 sweet potato
2 carrots
1 lime (peeled)

Clear Sky

Ingredients:

1 cucumber
1 green apple
1 zucchini
a cup of fresh blueberries
a cup of fresh blackberries
1 lime (peeled)
a bunch of fresh mint leaves

Dream

Ingredients:

1 cucumber
1 melon (peeled)
1 Kale
2 apples
a bunch of fresh mint

Will

Ingredients:

1 yellow pepper
1 celery stick
1 broccoli head
2 carrots
1 lemon (peeled)

Power

Ingredients:

1 pepper
1 zucchini
1 read cabbage
2 carrots
1 lemon (peeled)

Success

Ingredients:

1 lettuce
2 pears
2 kiwis (peeled)
2 celery sticks
1 lemon (peeled)

Garden Delight

Ingredients:

1 cucumber
2 oranges (peeled)
1 cabbage
2 carrots
1 lemon (peeled)

Triple C Booster

Ingredients:

2 kiwis (peeled)
1 celery stick
1 cucumber
2 apples
1 lemon (peeled)

Granny's little secret

Ingredients:

1 cucumber
1 red onion
4 white asparagus
a bunch of fresh coriander
1 lemon (peeled)

I yam what I yam

Ingredients:

1 cucumber
1 kale
a good bunch of fresh spinaches
1 lemon (peeled)
mint leaves

Powerful thoughts

Ingredients:

1 fennel bulb
3 carrots
1 red apple
1 lemon (peeled)
Sprinkle with cinnamon powder (optional)

Infinite supply

Ingredients:

3 parsnips
1 red pepper
1 celery stick
2 carrots
1 apple

Magnetic love

Ingredients:

½ cucumber
2 red peppers
2 carrots
1 green apple
1 broccoli head
½ lemon (peeled)
a teaspoon of curry powder (optional)

Open arms

Ingredients:

1 kale
a bunch of fresh chard
2 celery sticks
2 pears
3 carrots
1 lemon (peeled)

More goodness

Ingredients:

½ cucumber
1 eggplant
1 celery stick
2 carrots
2 apples
½ lemon (peeled)

Reward my commitment

Ingredients:

1 cucumber
1 celery stick
2 apples
2 radish
a tinny bit of fresh ginger root

Waterfalls

Ingredients:

½ watermelon (rind removed)
½ pineapple (peeled)
½ cucumber
1 orange (peeled)

Letting go

Ingredients:

1 melon (peeled)
1 celery stick
2 carrots
1 lemon (peeled)

Absolute Faith

Ingredients:

1 cucumber
1 celery stick
1 white onion
1 garlic clove
1 broccoli head
1 apple
1/2 lemon (peeled)

Blessed trust

Ingredients:

1 /2 cucumber
1 large tomato
2 apples
a little piece of fresh ginger root
a fresh bunch of parsley

Liquid gold

Ingredients:

1 cucumber
1 grapefruit (peeled)
1 sweet potato
1 apple
½ lemon (peeled)

Baby boom

Ingredients:

1 cucumber
1 melon (peeled)
2 pears
1 sweet potato
1 lime (peeled)

Self Confidence

Ingredients:

1 cucumber
a cup of fresh blueberries
2 apples
1 lemon (peeled)

Sense of purpose

Ingredients:

½ cucumber
1 turnip
4 carrots
2 apples
½ lemon (peeled)

Enthusiasm

Ingredients:

1 cucumber
1 parsnip
1 celery stick
2 pears
A bunch of fresh spinach
1 lime (peeled)

Expertise

Ingredients:

1 cucumber
1 cauliflower
1 red pepper
2 carrots
1 apple
1 lemon (peeled)

Preparation

Ingredients:

1 cucumber
1 broccoli head
1 celery stick
1 apple
1 lemon (peeled)

Self Reliance

Ingredients:

1 cucumber
4 carrots
a bunch of fresh spinach
1 apple
1 lemon (peeled)

Self Image

Ingredients:

1 cucumber
1 cabbage
2 celery sticks
2 green apples
2 carrots
a small piece of fresh ginger root

Charisma

Ingredients:

1 beetroot
2 carrots
1 sweet potato
1 radish
1 red apple

Self Discipline

Ingredients:

1 cucumber
1 beetroot
½ fennel bulb
2 apples
1 orange (peeled)

Extraordinary performance

Ingredients:

1 beetroot
1 sweet potato
1 tomato
1 apple
1 lemon (peeled)

Bipolar world

Ingredients:

1 cucumber
1 broccoli head
1 red pepper
1 red apple
1 lemon (peeled)

Persistence

Ingredients:

1 cucumber
1 kale
1 broccoli head
3 carrots
2 apples
1 lemon (peeled)

Live

Ingredients:

1 cucumber
2 radish
2 sweet potatoes
20 grapes
1 lime (peeled)

Laugh

Ingredients:

1 cucumber
2 sweet potatoes
1 red onion
2 carrots
1 lemon (peeled)

Love

Ingredients:

1 cucumber
1 orange (peeled)
1 broccoli head
a bunch of fresh mint leaves

Dance

Ingredients:

1 cucumber
4 plums (seedless)
2 peaches (seedless)
2 apricots (seedless)
1 apple

Give

Ingredients:

1 cucumber
2 oranges (peeled)
1 papaya (peeled)
1 lime (peeled)

Gratitude

Ingredients:

1 cucumber
2 kiwis (peeled)
3 pears

Evolve

Ingredients:

1 cucumber
3 carrots
1 melon (peeled)
2 nectarines (seedless)

Create

Ingredients:

1 cucumber
20 strawberries
2 apples
1 lime (peeled)

Smile

Ingredients:

1 cucumber
1 watermelon
2 oranges (peeled)

Love Silence

Ingredients:

1 cucumber
2 apples
20 black grapes
a cup of blueberries

Listen

Ingredients:

1 sweet potato
2 pears
2 oranges (peeled)

Act

Ingredients:

1 cucumber
The seeds of 1 pomegranate
2 pears

Learn

Ingredients:

1 cucumber
1 grapefruit (peeled)
1 sweet potato
1 orange

Do

Ingredients:

1 cup blueberries
1 cup blackberries
1 cup raspberries
1 cup strawberries

My dear juicing newbie,

What makes you a winner is rising above the circumstances no matter what.

If circumstances beat you is only because you let them!
This life is about consciousness and perseverance. It
is about dreaming, believing and taking guided actions
towards those dreams. And sometimes you have to
believe you can do it before you even do it.

I would like at this point to congratulate you for choos-
ing to get this book and no other. Believe there was a
reason for that!

You came to this book because you wanted to learn, to
get something out of this experience, a hidden message
among these simple lines. It is your juicer and this
is an investment that you have made to yourself. An
investment to your development towards unlocking your
true potential. So pat yourself on the back for taking the
decision to become a healthier and stronger version of
you and Welcome to the world of juicing!

With Love (because is all there is),

Ana Ortega

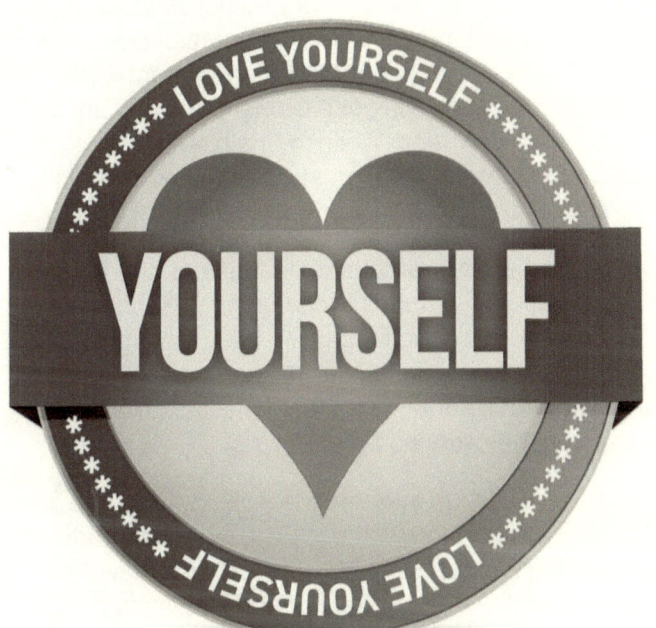

ABOUT THE AUTHOR

Ana Ortega (1980 -) is a writer and philosopher of New Thought who was born in the south of Spain. Her peasant parents taught her the value of hard work, perseverance and loving one's neighbour, and instilled in her a love of writing. While in Spain, Ana studied Audiovisual Communication and worked as a freelance newspaper columnist.

She spent her early adulthood in England, the United States and Latin America, working in marketing and becoming a seasoned financier. In this most productive stage of her professional life, she served as a consultant, communicator and finance professional, while continuing her work as a writer.

Currently, Ana is an internationally recognized Life Coach, who lives and works in Switzerland. In addition to writing and continuing her research into New Age philosophy, she teaches courses that have led to her being considered an expert in the philosophy of new thinking and she has hundreds of thousands of followers around the world.

Please send comments and suggestions to ana@anaortega.org.

Follow the healthy adventures of the author on Twitter: @DanaManana

Website: http://www.anaortega.org

Other works by
Ana Ortega

Vegan Recipes for Newbies
ISBN -1484072022

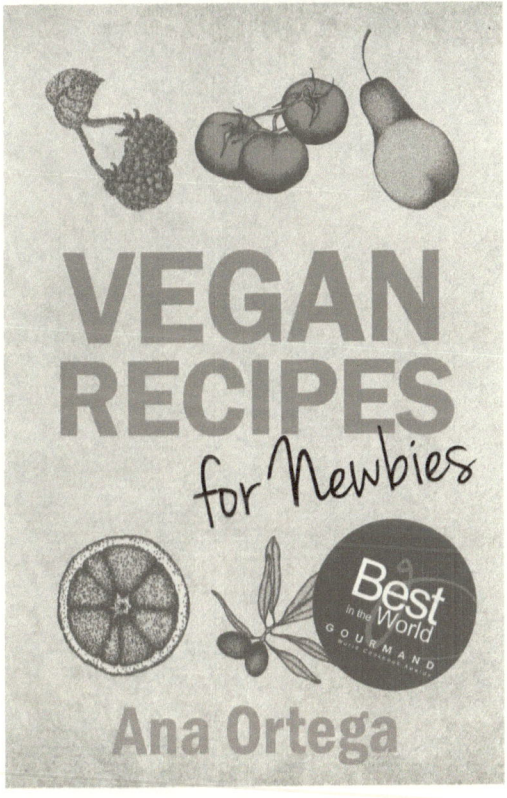

WINNER GOURMAND WORLD COOKBOOK AWARDS
2013 Category- Best Vegetarian Cookbook in the world

Taxi, Life Stories

ISBN -1500425125

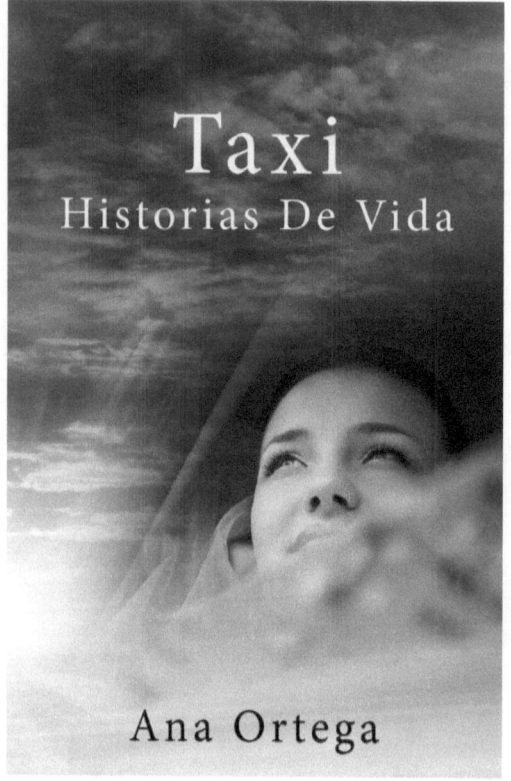

Taxi
Historias De Vida

Ana Ortega